INTERMITTENT FASTING

FOR WOMEN OVER 50

*The Ultimate Guide To Unlock The Secrets
To A Long And Healthy Lifestyle. Detox Your Body,
Lose Weight, Reset Metabolism,
Increase Your Energy, Delay Aging
And Rejuvenate Yourself*

Catherine Logan

CATHERINE LOGAN

Table of Contents

INTRODUCTION 8

CHAPTER 1: WHAT IS INTERMITTENT FASTING (IF)? 10

INTERMITTENT FASTING.. 10

SCIENCE BEHIND INTERMITTENT FASTING 12

WHAT HAPPENS WHEN YOU FAST? 13

MORE SCIENTIFIC DATA 16

CHAPTER 2: AUTOPHAGY **20**

AUTOPHAGY AND HOW DOES IT WORK.................................. 20

THE SCIENCE BEHIND AUTOPHAGY.. 22

THE BENEFITS.. 23

HOW TO ACTIVATE AUTOPHAGY 25

CHAPTER 3: PROS AND CONS OF INTERMITTENT FASTING .28

PROS 28

CONS... 31

CHAPTER 4: INTERMITTENT FASTING FOR WOMEN OVER 50

....**34**

CHANGES IN OUR BODIES AFTER THE AGE OF 50 34

HOW TO TAKE CARE OF YOUR BODY AFTER 50 37

BENEFITS OF INTERMITTENT FASTING ON WOMEN OVER 50 40

CHECK YOUR HORMONES 44

CHAPTER 5: TYPES OF INTERMITTENT FASTING **46**

THE 16:8 METHOD.. 46

THE 5:2 METHOD.. 48

ALTERNATE-DAY FASTING (ADF)..50

EAT-STOP-EAT 51

1 MEAL A DAY (OMAD) 52

THE WARRIOR DIET 53

CHAPTER 6: HOW TO START **56**

CREATE A MONTHLY CALENDAR 56

RECORD YOUR FINDINGS 56

PLAN YOUR MEALS..57

REWARD YOURSELF..58

CURB HUNGER PAINS...59

STAY BUSY..59

PRACTICE MINDFUL EATING 59

PRACTICE PORTION CONTROL..61

GET TECH SAVVY 62

LIFE FASTING TRACKER..62

MAKING THE CHANGE 63

WHEN TO START? 63

MEASURE YOUR EATING 63

KEEP UP YOUR EXERCISE PLAN 63

STOP, START, STOP 64

DO YOUR RESEARCH 64

HAVE FUN...64

KNOW YOUR BMI 65

HOW TO CALCULATE YOUR BMI 65

CHAPTER 7: DOS AND DON'TS ABOUT INTERMITTENT

FASTING...**68**

THE DOS 68

THE DON'TS..76

CHAPTER 8: COMMON MISTAKES 78

LOOKING FOR RESULTS TOO FAST...............79

CONFUSING THIRST WITH HUNGER 80

EATING UNHEALTHY FOODS..............81

TRYING TO STICK TO THE WRONG PLAN..............84

WORKING OUT TOO MUCH OR TOO LITTLE..............84

MISUNDERSTANDING REAL HUNGER SIGNS..............85

USING INTERMITTENT FASTING AS A JUSTIFICATION TO OVEREAT..............86

NOT EATING ENOUGH..............87

FAILING TO PLAN YOUR MEALS IN ADVANCE..............88

PERSEVERANCE IS THE KEY..............88

DON'T FRAME UNREALISTIC EXPECTATIONS..............89

CHAPTER 9: WHAT TO EAT AND WHAT TO AVOID 90

WHAT TO EAT..............90

WHAT TO AVOID..............93

INTERMITTENT FASTING AND THE KETO DIET..............95

CHAPTER 10: MAINTAINING WEIGHT 98

WHAT IS WATER WEIGHT? 98

WHAT LEADS TO THE LOSS OF WATER WEIGHT? 99

WHY CALORIE RESTRICTION IS INEFFECTIVE IN ACTUAL WEIGHT LOSS....101

THE REASON FOR WEIGHT RELAPSE..............103

CLEAN FOOD FOR A CLEAN MINDSET..............103

CHAPTER 11: MYTHS ABOUT INTERMITTENT FASTING 106

YOUR BODY WILL GO INTO STARVATION MODE AND METABOLISM WILL SLOW DOWN..............106

YOU'LL LOSE MUSCLE..............106

YOU'LL CERTAINLY INDULGE DURING EATING WINDOWS..............107

THERE'S JUST A SINGLE METHOD TO DO IF.................................107

YOU'LL BECOME EXTREMELY HEALTHY AND FIT BY FASTING 107

IT'S FOR EVERYONE...108

CHAPTER 12: HOW TO STAY MOTIVATED **110**

GET AN ACCOUNTABILITY PARTNER...110

KEEP INFORMED...111

SET GOALS WITH REWARDS 111

CONCENTRATE ON POSITIVE FEELINGS...112

HEALTHY-EATING MIND..113

VISUALIZE THE FUTURE 113

JOIN A COMMUNITY OF LIKE MINDS...114

CONCLUSION **116**

INTRODUCTION

A re you tired of trying different types of diets and not seeing results? Are you tired of dietary restrictions and sacrifices that you cannot commit to in the long run? Well, if the answer is yes then this is the book for you. We will explore what intermittent fasting is, how to get started, benefits, tips to follow, and how intermittent fasting can help you transform your life by adopting a healthier lifestyle.

Entering our 50s can be really challenging as our body starts to change and the small issues that we have been ignoring before start to affect our everyday lives. Hormonal issues appear, the immune system starts to fail and it is becoming increasingly difficult to lose weight especially in areas such as hips, belly, and love handles. Intermittent fasting is here to help. It is an effective and efficient way to stay fit and healthy. The different types of intermittent fasting allow us to find the one that better suits us based on our needs and busy lives. Intermittent fasting is not a diet but rather a habit and a lifestyle. It is all about when you eat. It is an eating pattern that helps you divide your day into periods of fasting and eating. It doesn't specify which foods you should eat but rather when you should eat them. In the 1980s counting calories was the only thing that mattered. Everyone, including myself, was so obsessed that we were carrying around a pocket-sized calorie counting book trying to calculate and sum up the calories of each meal. Advises from friends such as eat less or exercise more simply did not work. With intermittent fasting, you can reset your metabolism, lose weight, and rejuvenate the body. You don't have to cut calories or nutrients but, instead, you get all the nutrients that you need during your eating period and maintain your weight without exhausting diets thanks to intermittent fasting. The basics of healthy nutrition such as fresh fruits and vegetables, good fat and fiber, lean proteins still hold true, and if you want to see the benefits of intermittent fasting you should maintain good nutrition. It does take a mindset for intermittent fasting and there is no one-size-fits-all approach.

I hope you will find this book of value and will help you start your journey.

You got this!

Happy reading!

CHAPTER 1:

WHAT IS INTERMITTENT FASTING (IF)?

Intermittent Fasting

O therwise known as IF, is an eating pattern where you alternate periods of fasting and eating. It is all about when you eat and not what you eat. During these fasting periods, you don't eat anything besides water, herbal tea, coffee, or zero-calorie beverages. Within the eating window, you can fit in 2, 3, or more meals. For example, if you finish your last meal at 8 p.m. and don't eat until noon the next day, you're technically fasting for 16 hours. This works great for breakfast skippers. But if you are a breakfast person you can finish your last meal earlier and have breakfast slightly later in the morning. Even though you don't have to count calories during your eating window it is important to eat healthy foods because eating junk food can lead to a consumption of excessive calories. IF is not a new idea; it has been utilized in medical practice for over 2,000 years.

Fasting has been used for medicinal purposes since ancient times. Ancient Chinese medicine promoted the fasting of food before surgery in order to preserve energy and warded off evil spirits who may accompany physical ailments. Others, like the Egyptians, believed that fasting was a method for self-cleansing and purification. The goal was to rid both body and soul of harmful elements that may be holding back the person from performing their best. Dr. Sushruta the ancient Indian physician, known today as the father of Indian medicine, describes how intense meditation during a fast can lead to visions of religious figures, altered states of consciousness, enlightenment, or even mystical experiences. Fasting was seen as a method of developing self-control and gaining spiritual powers. Hippocrates, the father of Western medicine, believed fasting enabled the body to heal itself. He wrote, "To eat when you are sick, is to feed your illness." Plato, Socrates, and Aristotle all praised fasting. Paramahansa Yogananda, an Indian monk, yogi, and guru who introduced people to meditation said "Fasting is a natural method of healing." Dr. Herbert Shelton, the founder of the modern-day Natural Hygiene Health Movement, who supervised over 40,000 fasts, discusses in his books all the benefits of fasting for chronic diseases, including arthritis, heart disease, and more. Dr. Shelton wrote, "Fasting must be recognized as a fundamental and radical process that is older than any other mode of caring for the sick organism, for it is employed on the plane of instinct."

So, fasting is truly an idea that has survived the test of time.

Science Behind Intermittent Fasting

Let's put one thing upfront before we plunge into science: there isn't one way to do IF. The different types are described in detail in a later chapter, but what is important to understand at this point is that all types of IF are based on the same idea: The body can use its stored fat for energy to limit your caloric intake. Time-restricted eating offers more time for our body to use up fat. The goal is to systematically starve the body long enough to trigger fat burning.

So, how does our body fuel itself? It has 3 types of fuel: carbohydrates, fats, and proteins. It uses carbohydrates first, then fats, and finally uses protein if no other options are present.

Carbohydrates are broken down into glucose, the body's principal source of energy. So, when we eat, glucose can be used immediately as fuel or can be sent to the liver and stored as glycogen or fat.

Our body continues to function on glucose for a few hours from the carbohydrates we've just consumed. Typically, an inactive person takes about 10–12 hours to use up the glycogen stores, although someone that exercises may do so in less time. Once the glycogen reserves in the liver are depleted the body taps into its energy stores. This is when fats are broken down into fatty acids which are then converted into additional metabolic fuel. So, if we fast for longer periods the body starts to burn fat already stored and that's how we lose the extra fat.

But the moment we consume food again, even if it's just coffee with a bit of sugar and milk, we turn back to the previous mode and start burning carbohydrates and storing glycogen and fat. So, if you finish eating your evening snack at 10 p.m., your body will run out of glycogen at about 8 a.m. and start burning fat. If you normally eat breakfast at 8 a.m., but you change it to 11 a.m., you've given your body 3 extra hours to burn fat as fuel.

What Happens When You Fast?

Fasting begins about 8 hours after your last meal after which the liver will use the last of its glucose reserves and the body will start transitioning into fasting mode. As your blood glucose levels drop you might experience dizziness or drowsiness. Usually, these symptoms disappear as your body adjusts and you become used to fasting. However, if these symptoms persist and you cannot function properly you should stop fasting immediately.

Between 12–18 hours, your body has already exhausted the glucose and you've entered the metabolic state of ketosis in which there is a high concentration of ketones in the blood. Ketones are a type of chemical that your liver produces and your body uses them to start burning fat. And this is the secret to weight loss! One paradox with fasting is that it gets easier as you fast for a longer time and this is happening because ketones suppress appetite. Other benefits of an increased number of ketones include increased energy and better mood.

When you reach 24 hours, the body goes into a repair mode and begins to recycle old and damaged cells. This process is called autophagy and it has anti-aging and anti-inflammatory benefits. If you want to learn more about this powerful process and how it works then keep reading.

By the time you reach 48 hours without calories or with only a few calories, carbs, or protein, your growth hormone level is up to 5 times as high as when you started your fast. Increased HGH (Human Growth Hormone) level stimulates muscle repair and reduces fat tissue accumulation a very important process particularly as we age.

By 54 hours, your insulin has dropped to its lowest level point since you started fasting. Why is this a good thing? Insulin is a hormone made in the pancreas that regulates blood glucose. When we eat, insulin levels go up, it is then released into our bloodstream and our body starts to store fat. When we fast, insulin levels drop and our fat cells can then release their stored sugar, to be used as energy. To put it simply, the more we eat, the more insulin we produce and the more fat we store.

Constant high insulin levels may cause insulin insensitivity which in turn can cause prediabetes and diabetes type 2. Fasting helps to keep insulin levels low reducing diabetes risk.

In the final stage where you reach 72 hours of fasting, studies claim that your entire immune system can be regenerated. Your body is breaking down old cells and generating new ones. Starving the body can produce new white blood cells, which fight off infections. Please keep in mind that 72 hours without eating is a lot and needs to be done safely. Long-term fasts are not recommended for most people and should only be performed under medical supervision.

Now that you understand each stage your body goes through when you fast, it is time to break your fast and enter the refeeding stage! Cannot stress it enough but it's important to break your fast with a nutritious and balanced meal that will further improve the function of cells and tissues that went through cleanup while you were fasting.

Include plenty of vegetables, plant fibers and fats, proteins, and some whole grains. Avoid simple sugars and processed foods. Learn what works best for your body and enjoy the benefits of fasting.

More Scientific Data

Satchidananda Panda a professor of circadian biology at La Jolla, California's Salk Institute for Biological Studies, spent his career researching the human body's complex biochemical processes. His research in mice and individuals suggests that IF may improve human health in several different ways, including weight loss.

A 2012 research that Panda and his colleagues did with mice first suggested this. They took two genetically alike groups of mice and fed them the same diet. One group had access to the food for 24 hours, and the other group had access to it for only 8 hours.

The mice that were allowed to feed at all hours showed signs of insulin resistance after 18 weeks and had liver damage. But there were no such conditions for the mice that fed in the 8-hour window. They also weighed 28% less than mice with 24-hour food access, although the same number of calories were consumed a day by both groups of mice. "It was sort of earth-shattering," recalls Panda.

In recent years, scientists have discovered that so many of the human body's processes are linked to our circadian rhythms. For instance, most of us know that getting sunlight early in the morning is beneficial to our mood and sleep and that exposure to light at 9 p.m. via our mobile phones or laptops will interrupt our night's sleep. "Similarly, eating at the right time can nurture us, and healthy food at the wrong time can be junk food," says Panda. It is processed as fat instead of fuel, which makes sense if you analyze the fundamentals of how human metabolism functions.

Panda followed up on his time-restricted eating experiment in humans. In 2015, he and his colleagues put a small group of individuals on a time-restricted eating plan for 16 weeks. Interestingly, the researchers offered no diet instructions or advice at all to these individuals. Instead, the subjects were told to select a window of 10–12 hours to do all their feeding. The subjects displayed a small amount of weight loss after 16 weeks—an average of just over 8 pounds each. But according to Panda, they reported having better sleep, more energy in the mornings, and less hunger at bedtime, implying that time-restricted eating "actually has a systemic impact throughout the body."

In a study of 15 men at risk for type 2 diabetes conducted by Panda, he and his team found that after 1 week of limiting them to eating within a 9-hour window, the men exhibited a lower spike in blood glucose after a test meal, a sign of increased insulin sensitivity. It could help lower cholesterol as well. Panda and colleagues had 19 individuals in another trial, most of whom were on medication to reduce cholesterol or blood pressure or treat diabetes. They lowered their overall cholesterol by an average of around 11% after 12 weeks of eating within a 10-hour window.

Here is how you can practice time-restricted eating, according to Panda. Although some IF plans allow people to have unlimited amounts of coffee and tea during the day, he says that you should drink only water throughout your fasting window. This signifies no coffee, tea, or herbal tea, all of which can alter the blood's chemistry, which is why medical blood tests are not permitted during fasts.

Panda suggests drinking plain hot water after you wake up; it can give you some of the same calming feelings as coffee. Of course, he says it's OK to have some black coffee if it's necessary for you to be alert in the morning but stay away from any additional creamer, honey, sugar, or other sweeteners. "Only 1 teaspoon of sugar is enough to double our blood sugar," he says, which switches the body back into carb-burning mode and out of fat-burning mode.

Panda suggests that you wait until you've been up for a few hours to eat breakfast. The hormone cortisol spikes and high levels of cortisol will hinder your glucose regulation approximately 45 minutes after you wake up. Plus, the hormone melatonin, which makes our body ready for sleep, wears off about 2 hours after waking. This implies that your pancreas, which generates the insulin required to use carbohydrates in the food, is just only waking up for those first

2 hours. You should then try to finish your last meal about 2–3 hours before bedtime because that's when melatonin starts to prepare your body, as well as your pancreas, for sleep.

CHAPTER 2:

AUTOPHAGY

W hat if there is a way to stay forever young? What if you could erase a couple of years from your face and skin and take off some inches from your waistline by activating an internal cleanup process? Would you not want to know how to do that? Well, staying forever young or finding a fountain of youth might be unlikely but you can stimulate a natural process to keep cells rejuvenated and functioning optimally for the rest of your life. That process is known as autophagy.

Autophagy and How Does It Work

Reduce, reuse, and recycle is a popular phrase you're likely to hear in discussions about environmental sustainability. This is comparable in numerous ways to what autophagy does—reducing or breaking down and repairing parts of your cells and then recycling important body chemicals that can be reused by the liver.

In a nutshell, autophagy is the natural process that removes toxic materials and broken cells from your body to create new and healthier cells. The term comes from Latin which translates to self-eating (auto = "self" and phagy = "to eat"). In a weird way, this means your body is eating itself! Don't panic, it's a good thing. It's a rejuvenation process for your body.

If you fully realize what autophagy is and how to make it work for you, you will want to find ways to consciously stimulate the process because it can keep you feeling and looking younger than your real age! Older adults, in particular, can use this natural process to increase longevity.

Here's a simple analogy of how autophagy works that I think a lot of people can relate to. Think of what happens inside your kitchen when you are preparing a delicious meal. You are creating something heartfelt and delicious while at the same time making a mess and producing waste. If you leave your kitchen dirty after preparing your meal, it will be difficult to make your next meal. So, you do what any decent people do: throw or put away leftovers, clean the counter, put away unused ingredients, and recycle some of the food if you can. This is exactly how autophagy works in your body. It cleans up after you!

A big mess is created each day inside the body. This mess includes parts of dead cells, damaged proteins, and harmful particles that prevent optimal body function. When you were much younger, the process of autophagy clears this mess up as quickly as possible, keeping you looking young and supple. But as you grow older, the cleanup process slows down. Dirt, mess, and crumbs start to build up internally. If left unattended, the buildup can result in rapid aging, increased risk of cancer and dementia, as well as other diseases associated with old age.

But growing older doesn't mean you're doomed to have an inefficient cellular cleaning process. You can stimulate the process of autophagy and make it work as it used to when you were a lot younger. A method to do that is by decreasing insulin levels and increasing your glucagon levels. In simpler terms, fast and go without food for longer than you usually would. When you get really hungry as you do when you fast, your glucagon is increased and stimulates autophagy.

You can achieve some positive life-altering benefits by simply activating autophagy. But before going into the immense health benefits, let us consider the science behind the process, albeit briefly.

The Science Behind Autophagy

Autophagy in humans is induced by the activation of a protein known as p62. As soon as broken or damaged cells caused by metabolic byproducts begin to appear, p62 stimulates the process of clearing up the clutter at a cellular level. All remaining parts of waste or damaged cells that can lead to health problems are reduced, reused, and recycled. Think of the process as decluttering at a cellular level. The entire process is neatly executed to keep you healthy, strong to handle any biological stress, and of course, keep you looking and feeling young.

Researchers from Newcastle University found that humans evolved to live longer by responding well to biological stressors (Newcastle University, 2018). Usually, fruit flies can't withstand stress. But when researchers genetically altered fruit flies by giving them the human version of p62, they found that the fruit flies lived longer than usual even under stressful conditions.

The Benefits

Some people are said to have different biological and chronological ages. That is to say, their age is different from the quality of their life. Women are more likely to worry about showing signs of aging or looking older than men. Thankfully, you can look younger by activating autophagy. What the process does to your cells is to remove toxins and recycle cells instead of creating new ones. These rejuvenated cells will behave like new and work better.

Your skin is constantly exposed to harmful lights, air, chemicals, as well as harsh weather conditions. This causes damage to your skin cells. As the damaged cells continue to accumulate, your skin begins to wrinkle, lose elasticity, and no longer appear smooth. The process of autophagy repairs your skin cells that might have been partly damaged to make your skin glow and healthier. In the same way that wear and tear happens with things you use frequently, wear and tear (microtear) also happen to your muscles as you use them, especially during exercises. Your muscles become inflamed and require repairs. What this means is you need more energy to use these specific muscles. The process of autophagy in your cells will degrade the damaged parts in the muscle, reduce the amount of energy sent to the muscle, and ensure energy balance.

To keep your metabolism working well, your cells need to be in top shape. The powerhouse of your cell is the mitochondria. A lot of harmful trash is left behind in the mitochondria as it performs its function of burning fat and making adenosine triphosphate (ATP)—the molecule that stores all the energy you need to do almost everything. This harmful trash can damage your cells. Autophagy ensures that these toxins are promptly taken care of to prevent damage to your cells and keep them in a healthy state.

Several processes and activities that occur during your cellular cleaning and repair also help you to maintain a healthy weight. For example, when toxins are removed from your cells through autophagy and you successfully excrete them, your fat cells can no longer store these toxins. Also, when you fast for short periods (12–16 hours), autophagy is activated, fat-burning also takes place, and since it is not a prolonged fast, your proteins are spared. All these activities and processes help to make you leaner and fitter.

The cells of your gastrointestinal tract hardly ever take breaks. You put them to work consistently, and this can affect digestive health. Autophagy helps repair and restore the cells. When you stop eating for long periods you give your gut ample time to rest and heal. Giving your gut some rest (from digesting your meal) is vital for overall improved digestive health.

Certain neurodegenerative illnesses, for example, Alzheimer's disease and Parkinson's disease are a result of too much accumulation of damaged proteins around the brain cells. Autophagy clears this clutter of damaged proteins that don't work as they should. Dementia is not a standard portion of aging, even though it is largely linked to older people. You can keep all these illnesses at bay by activating autophagy. If your brain cells are clear of clutter (damaged protein cells), you will perform cognitive functions optimally.

How to Activate Autophagy

As already stated, one of the quickest ways to activate autophagy is by staying away from food for longer periods. In other words, IF can create just the right level of stress on your body to kick start the internal cleanup process. Going without food leads to an energy deficit, and that induces autophagy ridding your body of decaying cells and accumulated junk. So, besides the widely known weight-loss benefits of IF, perhaps a far-reaching positive aspect of practicing IF is activating autophagy.

Physical exercise is another stress-inducing activity that can stimulate autophagy. This is predominantly true for parts of the body where the process of metabolic regulation occurs. Some of these areas of the body where exercise-induced autophagy occurs are the liver, muscles, and pancreas.

When you combine IF with moderate physical exercises, you are taking autophagy to a new level. And considering all the benefits that you get from autophagy, isn't it worth giving up snacking after dinner?

CHAPTER 3:

PROS AND CONS OF INTERMITTENT FASTING

E ach dietary plan has its own pros and cons and you should know about the benefits and challenges before making a decision.

Pros

Simple to Follow

Numerous dietary examples center on eating specific nutrients and restricting or keeping away from different food sources. Learning the particular standards of an eating style can require significant time. For instance, there are whole books committed to understanding the DASH diet or figuring out how to follow a Mediterranean-style diet plan. With IF, you just eat as indicated by the hour of day or day of the week. When you've figured out which IF method is best for you, all you need is a watch or a schedule to remind yourself when to eat.

No Calorie Counting

As anyone might expect, following a normal diet requires you to count calories, and most of the time you should also stay away from them. Fortunately, with IF you don't have to worry about that anymore. You can still consume the same amount of calories and enjoy your favorite foods.

A study in 2011 found that individuals are bound to follow diet plans when someone else provides to them already made weekly or monthly meal plans and sometimes precooked meals. Commercial eating diets, WW, Jenny Craig, and others offer these services but not free of charge. However, many people don't have the assets to pay for these already prepared meal plans as they can be very expensive. With IF, practically no calorie-checking is required.

No Macronutrient Limitations

There are well-known eating plans that practically exclude the consumption of specific macronutrients. For instance, numerous people follow a low-carb diet to support well-being or get in shape. Others follow a low-fat diet for therapeutic or weight loss purposes. Every one of these approaches requires going to shop to embrace another eating method—regularly replacing most loved nourishments with new and perhaps new food sources. This may require new cooking abilities and figuring out how to shop and unexpectedly stock the kitchen.

None of these abilities are required with IF and there is absolutely no need to exclude specific macronutrients.

Unrestricted Eating

Anyone who has ever changed their eating routine to accomplish a health advantage or arrive at a stable weight realizes that you begin to desire foods that you are advised not to eat. With IF food limitation just happens during certain hours. On the non-fasting hours or days, you can generally eat anything you desire.

Boosts Longevity

One of the most broadly referred advantages of IF includes life span. As indicated by the National Institute on Aging, rat examines have demonstrated that when mice are put on projects that seriously confine calories (regularly during fasting periods) many showed an augmentation of life expectancy and diminished paces of a few ailments, particularly malignant growths. So, does this advantage extend to people too? According to studies, it does. As indicated by a survey distributed in 2010, there have been research findings that connect fasting to long-haul life span benefits.

Advances Weight Loss

Different human studies have shown that people who follow an IF plan manage to lose weight. Fasting each day for a period of time promotes calorie restriction and leads to weight loss. Also compared to calorie restriction diets, IF with sufficient protein intake and resistance training improves fat loss while also retaining fat-free mass which is basically our muscle mass.

Helps to Control Glucose and Cholesterol

Insulin resistance is thought to be a major cause of type 2 diabetes. Studies suggest that IF may improve insulin sensitivity and glucose homeostasis. Also, IF may help to improve LDL and cholesterol levels. Some research has also shown that it may reduce blood pressure and triglyceride levels. Additionally, it has been linked to reducing inflammation in the body and improving conditions associated with inflammation such as Alzheimer's disease, arthritis, and asthma. That reduction can happen because of a reduction in blood cells that cause inflammation—called "monocytes" when you fast.

Cons

Low Energy levels

Studies exploring the advantages of IF also point to specific symptoms during the fasting phase.

For instance, it isn't unusual to feel irritable, tired, experience headaches, and lack energy when your calories are minimal. Our bodies need fuel to maintain our energy levels to go through the day and some people will find practicing IF challenging with the lack of fuel. In this case, you might want to try fasting on a day of the week or period of time that you don't need to be very active. Even though IF is considered to be safe, it's not for everyone. If you have gastroesophageal reflux, diabetes, or other medical problems, talk with your doctor before starting any IF plan.

Extreme Hunger

As anyone might expect, it is normal for those in the fasting phase to encounter an uncomfortable hunger feeling. You may start to experience hunger pangs, or "hanger" which translates into feeling hungry and angry. Usually, if you manage to get through the first 20 minutes then it gets better.

Medications

You have to be very mindful when you take meds. A few meds explicitly state that they ought to be taken with food. Hence, taking meds during fasting might be a test. Anyone who is on medication should consult with their doctor before beginning IF, to ensure that the fasting stage won't meddle with the prescription's viability or will not worsen symptoms.

No Focus on Nutritious Eating

Just because IF is based on timing rather than food restriction it does not mean that during your eating window you can eat unhealthy meals, sweets, and cakes. Try to maintain a healthy diet that consists of fresh fruits and vegetables, lean protein foods, and whole-grain food. Of course, you can treat yourself to something sweet or have a glass of wine but make sure not to overdo it.

May Promote Overeating

As discussed, because IF can lead to increased hunger this, in turn, can lead to binge eating and overeating, which in turn can leave you bloated and filled with eater's remorse. Do not panic and resume your regular plan as soon as possible. Try to increase your exercise and drink lots of water.

Might Interfere With Your Social Eating

Eating together is an important aspect of our lives. It is a way to meet with friends and family, celebrate events, and spend time with the people we love. It is also a very important aspect of our working life as a lot of times we have to attend lunch business meetings or even celebrate important events. IF might interfere with your social eating activities since you only have a very small window to eat. Do not panic and make a plan. Socialize more than you eat. Think about your food options and pick one with fewer calories. Be mindful of how many drinks you will have and consider mixing them with water.

CHAPTER 4:

INTERMITTENT FASTING FOR WOMEN OVER 50

Changes in Our Bodies After the Age of 50

So, you have reached the age of 50 and you notice that every day your body changes and hormones "go crazy." The well-formed body of 30 is lost—that is true. The body you had in your 20s, 30s, or 40s will probably not come back, but think about what it took for this body to get here today: probably 1 or more pregnancies, stress, anxiety about everyday life, and, of course, dealing with menopause.

These are some of the changes that you will encounter at this age:

Skin and Hair Changes

Your skin will start to become thinner and produce fewer natural oils, which will cause it to become drier and less elastic. The cells in the scalp will begin to produce less pigment causing the hairs to shrink and turn white.

Vision and Hearing Changes

Decreased vision and hearing are a natural consequence of aging. Many of us need reading glasses, as it becomes difficult for the eyes to focus on nearby objects. Hearing problems are also common as we age. It is something that happens gradually, so many times it is not perceived.

Changes in Sleep Patterns

The good news is that as we grow older, we need less sleep than younger people. The less good news is that we also tend to wake up more often during the night and not sleep as deeply as when we were younger.

Body Weight Changes

As you grow older, your body needs less energy. If you keep consuming the same amount of calories as when you were younger, you will gain weight. Muscle mass decreases with age and this will cause your metabolism to slow down which, in turn, will lead to getting a few extra pounds. Adding exercise to your routine can help and prevent gaining weight.

Heart Function Changes

Your heart rate slows with age and your arteries become harder. These 2 things can put pressure on your heart and your heart muscles can expand and as a result, many people develop heart disease.

Your Bones and Joints Changes

As with all things, long-term use of our bodies causes wear and tear. With age, you might develop osteoporosis, which reduces skeletal bone density. This could lead to bone fractures. Many people also lose weight from this cause. Osteoarthritis is also a common condition.

Bladder Control Changes

As muscle function declines so can bladder control. It can range from minor "leaks" to severe bladder control problems.

Brain Function Changes

The brain has the amazing ability to adapt to changing conditions and many people remain perceptive for the rest of their lives. But some might start experiencing gradual memory loss as they grow older. This can range from mild to severe and is sometimes a sign of the onset of Alzheimer's disease. With regular exercise and by constantly training your mind you can improve your cognitive function or even slow down the process.

However, the body can improve dramatically at any age as long as there are a method and routine. Below you will discover some ways that can improve not only the body after you turn 50 but also your psychology in relation to it.

How to Take Care of Your Body After 50

As in any age, proper nutrition and exercise are the most effective ways to prevent problems after turning 50 and to provide what your body needs. According to experts, these are the changes we need to make in our daily habits as we enter the 5th decade of our life:

Keep Exercising

Physical activity is scientifically proven to help women over 50. It maintains a high basic metabolic rhythm and helps maintain muscle mass and reduce fat. It also has a positive effect on the hormonal system by producing endorphins, the hormones that improve mood. Exercise helps prevent osteoporosis as it maintains bone density at normal levels. Another important benefit of exercise is that it reduces the symptoms of menopause like insomnia, irritability, and hot flashes.

Start Meditating

Meditation has a beneficial effect on the nervous system as it relieves stress and anxiety through concentration in the breath. At the same time, it improves the cardiorespiratory function as it slows down the heart rate, lowers blood pressure, and helps treat obesity because it increases the production of serotonin, a hormone that when low is associated with depression, obesity, insomnia, and headaches. In addition, it reduces the symptoms of menopause.

More Calcium for Bone Health

The risk of osteoporosis increases after menopause, with 1 in 3 women over 50 having an increased chance of fracturing, according to research. Although this problem affects some men, it is usually a woman's "privilege." The reason is that our body absorbs less calcium as we grow older, while at the same time increasing the chances of developing intolerance to dairy products which are the main source of calcium. Alternatively, we can get the calcium we need by eating vegetables with large green leaves (kale, lettuce, spinach, celery, etc.) or juices fortified with calcium. Estimate that a woman over 50 needs about 1,200 mg. per day to maintain her bone health.

More Protein for a Healthy Muscular System

Losing muscle mass is a normal process that occurs over time and is exacerbated by the fact that women over 50 usually lead a more sedentary lifestyle and exercise less. But if not treated in time, when we reach 80, we will have lost up to half the muscle mass. One of the main ways to avoid it is to provide the body with protein; its most important source is meat, but there are also plant sources, such as soy, quinoa, eggs, nuts, vegetables, and legumes. The amount of protein a woman needs depends on her body weight and is estimated at about 1–

1.5 g. per pound. For example, if you weigh 60 kg., you should consume 60–90 g. of protein.

Vitamin 12 for Brain Function

As we grow older, the body loses the ability to absorb nutrients as much as possible. One of the ingredients that is often not absorbed enough is vitamin B-12, which is essential for bones, blood vessels, and brain function. Its best sources are eggs, milk, lean meat, fish, and cereals that are fortified with B-12. You should pay even more attention if you are vegan, as B-12 deficiency is a problem that is often observed in those who follow a vegetarian diet. The amount a woman over 50 needs is 2.4 mg.—if you think you are not getting enough through your diet, it is advisable to discuss with your doctor the possibility of taking a supplement.

It is very important at this age to focus on a good and nutritious diet. Increase consumption of fruits and vegetables, drink fresh juices, eat legumes and cereals, as well as fish and seafood. Reduce consumption of sugar, alcohol, and red meat. Make sure you prepare your own meals and prioritize yourself and not just the care of others.

Benefits of Intermittent Fasting on Women over 50

Over the age of 50, it is increasingly difficult for a woman to lose weight and we are obsessed with those extra pounds that accumulate in areas where we do not want them to, such as hips and love handles. IF is an alternative to the usual diets, and can also become a way of life.

The different types of IF allow us to evaluate and choose the most suitable one for us, adapting it to our needs and lifestyle.

Obviously, it is necessary, as mentioned before, to maintain a balanced and healthy diet, rich in vegetables and whole grains and one that provides all the macronutrients needed by the body, as well as the right amount of fat (preferably vegetable) and avoid junk food, seasoned, and too salty. All in all, you can eat anything, even taking a few whims from time to time.

Fasting has positive implications for the health of women over 50. Science has shown that reducing calorie intake prolongs life, because it acts on the metabolic function of longevity genes, reduces senile diseases, cancer, cardiovascular diseases, and neurodegenerative ones such as Alzheimer's and Parkinson's disease. In addition, especially for women over 50, it has multiple benefits on mood, fights depression, and contributes to the improvement of energy, libido, and concentration. And as if these weren't enough, it gives the skin a better look.

To start this type of "diet" you must first of all be in good health and, in any case, before starting, it is always better to consult your doctor. The female body is particularly sensitive to calorie restriction, because the hypothalamus, a gland in the brain responsible for the production of hormones, is stimulated. These hormones risk going haywire with a drastic reduction in calories or too long on a fast. The advice is therefore to start gradually, perhaps introducing some vegetable snacks during fasting hours (fennel, lettuce, endive, radicchio).

As mentioned, in women, IF works differently than in men. Sometimes it is more difficult for women to get results. Physiological and weight benefits are still possible but sometimes require a different approach. In addition, IF on non-consecutive days is better able to keep those annoying hormones under control. Various scientific evidence shows that in order to achieve fat loss, fasting must be tailored to the sex.

For women, in particular, there are specific biological truths about fasting which, if you ignore them, will prevent you from achieving your goals of a better body and fitness. Fasting can really prove to be a convenient and effective way to optimize your health and make you feel better, but only if it is done in a certain way; the way that is best for each one of us.

Fasting, after all, represents the easiest and at the same time powerful detoxification and regeneration therapy that we can offer to cells and the whole organism. Putting certain functions at physiological rest does not, in fact, mean that organs and tissues go on stand-by. On the contrary, thanks to the absence of a continuous metabolic commitment, they can dedicate themselves to something else, activating all those processes of self-repair, catabolism, excretion, and cell turnover that only in the absence of nutrients can take place at the highest levels.

At the beginning, and especially the first few times, you don't realize what is happening inside, but it takes very little to feel the effects. Apart from the slight headache that can arise the first time, you usually feel more energetic, concentrated, and serene soon. Not only that, the perennial feeling of hunger turns into pleasant and constant satiety, which is maintained even after returning to normal nutrition.

Another effect of IF, especially in overweight women, is to be able—without too much difficulty—to lose weight in the form of adipose tissue. Compared to a chronic low-calorie diet, in fact, an IF protocol can be a much more feasible and effective approach. There are many cases of women who, after trying it, learn to eat well even on feeding days.

In normal-weight women, however, the effect on body composition is more unpredictable and controversial. There are those who expect to lose weight but are disappointed because the weight does not vary, and those who don't, notice better results.

In the first case, it is necessary to understand whether or not the desired weight loss was necessary at the outset, and especially if there are changes in body composition, which is much more important than weight itself. Weight loss, after all, should not be the first or only purpose of IF. Some women may also experience morphological changes in their body, such as a thinning waist or a reduction in hip circumference, and this is certainly related to hormonal factors as well as changes in glucidic and insulin metabolism (better insulin sensitivity, less tendency to accumulate visceral fat). These different reactions allow us to make a very important reflection, which concerns the differences between one woman and another in terms of body composition and location of accumulations. For this reason, we must, first of all, make it clear which objectives we want to achieve and understand that every woman is different from the other.

Each woman is characterized by her own personal type and endocrine profile, which determines a wide variability in terms of body composition, glucidic and lipid metabolism, and tendency to accumulate fat in localized areas. Some women, for example, store more adipose tissue at the abdominal level, while some others on thighs and buttocks.

It is clear, therefore, that it is useful to assess if IF and what type of IF is for you taking into consideration also your body type.

Check Your Hormones

Hormones can be easily thrown out of whack by the slightest change in her already established pattern of behavior. Whether it is a physical change such as altering your eating pattern or an emotional change such as being irritated or sad, it can bring about hormonal imbalance in a woman even if it is temporary.

But for perimenopausal and menopausal women, hormones can go haywire for reasons even they can't define. You could be feeling really great all week, and without anything changing you could suddenly become fatigued, depressed, and not in the right frame of mind. These changes happen due to the unpredictability of this phase of a woman's life. Because this can happen for no apparent reason, it is best to check your hormonal levels before putting your body through a major lifestyle change. If you've ever had issues with thyroid, cortisol, or adrenal fatigue, ensure that you have these checks before you begin.

This could be a surprise to some women, but your ovaries produce testosterone, too. So, as you grow older and begin to experience a decline in your estrogen and progesterone levels, your testosterone levels are also taking a nosedive. Your libido can be affected by low levels of testosterone and make you feel exhausted and bummed out for no reason at all. So, while you are checking your other hormones, don't forget to do a testosterone test. The thyroid and testosterone hormones also help in weight regulation. So, if you intend to shed some weight using IF, these tests are very necessary.

CHAPTER 5:

TYPES OF INTERMITTENT FASTING

A ll IF methods are beneficial and effective, but it depends on each individual to find out which one works better. Several types of IF exist. The most prominent ones are:

The 16:8 Method

One of the most popular methods of fasting for losing weight is the 16:8 IF plan. Basically, you fast for 16 hours and restrict eating to an 8-hour window of time.

Say you start eating at 10 a.m. you would then stop eating at 6 p.m. Or you could start eating at noon and eat till 8 p.m. Or you could start eating at 8 a.m. and be done eating at 4 p.m.

First of all, choose whether you're going to find it easier to skip dinner or you're going to find it's easier to skip breakfast. So, if you decide to skip breakfast, think, what time do you normally have your breakfast? The average person says 8 a.m. Then rather than 8 a.m., go into work or whatever you are doing and wait until 10 a.m. and see how you feel. And then basically, over the course of 2 weeks, push until it's a 16-hour gap.

Some people choose to miss dinner instead. You could restrict the eating window to 9 a.m. and 5 p.m. per day with this.

If you carefully choose the timing of meals, like breakfast at 10:00 a.m., lunch at 2:00 p.m., and dinner at 5:30 p.m. you can still enjoy all 3 main meals of the day. By 6:00 p.m. you can finish eating your dinner so that all of the food consumption is done inside the 10 a.m. to 6 p.m. window, which is 8 hours.

Whereas other diet plans can set rigid rules and regulations, the 16:8 process is more flexible and based on the time-restricted feeding (TRF) method. This is the best method to follow at least 3 days a week when your work or everyday schedule is not regular.

A study found that the 16:8 technique helped decrease body fat and maintained muscle mass in several participants when coupled with physical exercise. A much more recent study showed that the 16:8 method did not hinder muscle gains in women performing aerobic exercise.

While the 16:8 technique can easily fit into every lifestyle, it may be difficult for some individuals to avoid eating 16 hours straight. Additionally, the potential benefits associated with 16:8 IF can be negated by eating junk food or too many snacks during the 8-hour window. To maximize this intermittent fasting's health benefits, find out whatever works for your schedule but still try to get in all the right nutrients your body needs, make sure to eat a healthy, balanced diet containing fresh vegetables, fruits, whole grains, good lean protein, and healthy fats.

The 16:8 Method

Time Schedule	Monday	Tuesday	Wednesday	Thursday	Friday	Saturday	Sunday
Midnight 4 am 8 am	Fast	Fast	Fast	Fast	Fast	Fast	Fast
12 pm	First meal	First meal	First meal	First meal	First meal	First meal	First meal
4 pm	Last meal by 8 pm	Last meal by 8 pm	Last meal by 8 pm	Last meal by 8 pm	Last meal by 8 pm	Last meal by 8 pm	Last meal by 8 pm
8 pm Midnight	Fast	Fast	Fast	Fast	Fast	Fast	Fast

Schedule is indicative and can be adjusted based on your daily routine

The 5:2 Method

The 5:2 diet usually entails consuming normal amounts of calories 5 days each week while reducing your calorie consumption for only 2 days of the week. You can eat normally for 3 days and then fast for 1 day. Then you can eat normally for the next 2 days and fast for the 7th day. You can choose whichever 2 days of the week you prefer, as long as there is at least 1 non-fasting day in between them.

The 5:2 diet is simple and direct. You normally eat 5 days a week and don't limit your calories and then you drop the calorie consumption to ¼ of your standard requirements for the remaining 2 days of the same week. This means reducing the calorie intake to just 500 calories each day, 2 days per week, for someone who regularly consumes 2,000 calories each day.

As the person gets to select the days they are fasting, the 5:2 diet promises versatility, and there are no guidelines on whether or what to consume on full-calorie days. Having said that, it should be remembered that eating "usually" on full-calorie days does not grant you a free pass to consume anything you want. It is recommended that women consume 500 calories on fasting days. But since calorie intake is limited try to use your calories wisely. Focus on nutritious, high-fiber, high-protein foods that will make you feel full without consuming too many calories. Soups are also great options for fasting days. You can have 2 meals, lunch, and dinner of 250 calories each. Try yogurt with berries, grilled fish or boiled eggs, big portions of vegetables, and of course don't forget to drink as much water as you can. It's not easy to restrict oneself to only 500 calories a day, even though it's just 2 days a week. And, you can feel sick or faint from eating very few calories. The 5:2 diet might be efficient, but it's not for everybody. In order to see if the 5:2 diet could be appropriate for you, speak to the doctor. According to research, for people with type 2 diabetes, the 5:2 diet is as efficient as daily calorie reduction for weight loss and blood sugar control. Another study showed that the 5:2 diet for both weight reduction and the treatment of metabolic disorders such as cardiac failure and diabetes was almost as successful as constant calorie restriction.

Furthermore, cholesterol levels, blood pressure, and inflammation were decreased. All IF groups lost more body fat than the normal calorie restriction community. Just remember, when you follow any low-calorie diet, it's important to make every calorie work. This means choosing nutrient-dense foods. Don't blow your entire days' worth of calories on one slice of cake, please!

Alternate-Day Fasting (ADF)

It involves eating normally on some days and fasting on others, so you can get the best of both worlds: the health benefits of fasting and the positive effects that come with eating. The basic idea is that you fast on one day and then eat what you want the next day. On a day you're not fasting, eat as usual. On a day you're fasting, you take in only water (black coffee and tea are ok), or anything with less than 50 calories per serving.

If you're considering alternate day fasting, benefits include: It improves your energy levels and helps you lose weight and belly fat. Also, studies have shown lower levels of LDL cholesterol and increased ketone bodies.

Can a woman over 50 do it? Yes. Women who alternate daily with fasting and eating experience a decrease in estrogen levels, which helps to reduce the risk of breast cancer. Your body is also in a constant state of fat burning. And it doesn't matter if you're overweight or not, because you can lose weight by fasting on alternate days. Just keep in mind that a full fast every other day is rather extreme, so it's not recommended for beginners and you should consult with your doctor. You might experience low levels of energy and dehydration. Also, you should avoid ADF if you are taking medication as some medicines cannot be taken on an empty stomach. However, if you want to try it you can follow a modified ADF approach where you are allowed to eat about 500 calories on fasting days and has proved to be as effective.

Eat-Stop-Eat

Eat-stop-eat is a different approach to IF popularized by fasting expert Brad Pilon. With this approach, you fast for up to 2 non-consecutive days each week for a 24-hour cycle. Drinking plenty of water is essential but you're also allowed other types of calorie-free beverages, such as unsweetened or artificially sweetened coffee or tea. Keep in mind though, that drinks that contain artificial sweeteners can trigger cravings. You can eat freely during the remaining days of the week. The idea behind a 24-hour fast every week is that eating fewer calories will ultimately lead to weight loss. Fasting for 24 hours can result in a metabolic shift that causes one's body to utilize stored fat rather than glucose as an energy source. For example, if you normally consume 1,800 calories per day, following eat-stop-eat for 2 days a week results in a calorie deficit of $2 \times 1,800 = 3,600$ calories per week. The common advice has long been that you need to burn 3,500 more calories than you eat to drop one pound. Eat-stop-eat may seem similar to the 5:2 diet. However, there is a key difference. The 5:2 diet allows the intake of about 500 calories during the fasting days but with eat-stop-eat, you have to refrain from food for an entire 24-hour period. It requires a huge amount of self-discipline to avoid food for 24 hours and may lead to bingeing and excessive consumption on non-fasting days. It may also result in eating disordered patterns. Before attempting eat-stop-eat, speak with your doctor and see if that could be an appropriate weight reduction solution for you.

Method	Monday	Tuesday	Wednesday	Thursday	Friday	Saturday	Sunday
5:2	Eat	Fast 500 Calories	Eat	Eat	Fast 500 Calories	Eat	Eat
ADF	Eat	24 hour Fast or Eat very few hundred calories	Eat	24 hour Fast or Eat very few hundred calories	Eat	24 hour Fast or Eat very few hundred calories	Eat
Eat Stop Eat	Eat	24 hour Fast	Eat	Eat	24 hour Fast	Eat	Eat

1 Meal a Day (OMAD)

Eating one meal a day is a practice that many people swear by to lose weight and improve overall health. This means that a person spends 23 hours of the day fasting, leaving just 1 hour per day to consume calories. Eat at 7 p.m. on the first day, for example, and fast until 7 p.m. the following day. Conversely, a person can choose to eat earlier, either lunch or breakfast, and fast until the next day for 23 hours. This sort of fasting is usually performed once or twice a week, but it can be more frequently adopted. This is the ultimate type of IF, and for many individuals, it can be an effective strategy for extreme weight loss. This type of fasting is not for everyone though and, compared to other fasting methods, eating just once per day is extreme and may have side effects such as increased hunger or slow metabolism. Restraining from food for so many hours can lead to lightheadedness, nausea, hypoglycemia, and dehydration. You will probably miss out on various meals with family and friends. The main issue is that you are following rules instead of making choices and that's the opposite of cultivating a mindful eating practice.

One Meal a Day or OMAD

Time Schedule	Monday	Tuesday	Wednesday	Thursday	Friday	Saturday	Sunday
Midnight 4 am 12 pm	Fast	Fast	Fast	Fast	Fast	Fast	Fast
12 pm	First meal	First meal	First meal	First meal	First meal	First meal	First meal
13 pm Midnight	Fast	Fast	Fast	Fast	Fast	Fast	Fast

Schedule is indicative and can be adjusted based on your daily routine

The Warrior Diet

This IF plan is called the warrior diet based on ancient warriors' eating patterns. The warrior diet, which was created in 2001, is a bit more dramatic than the 16:8 techniques but less rigid than the eat-stop-eat method. It comprises eating almost nothing or very little for 20 hours during the day and overnight, then eating as much food as desired in the evening in a 4-hour eating window.

The warrior diet consists of 3 phases for 3 weeks:

- **Week 1.** The 1st week is detox week. In the 20-hour period, you are allowed to eat hard-boiled eggs, vegetables and fruits, cheese and yogurt, broth, coffee, tea, and of course plenty of water. In the 4-hour eating window, you can eat salads and add some oil or vinegar and consume plant-based foods such as beans and whole grains such as quinoa, rice, bulgur, and oatmeal. The target is to remove toxins from the body.
- **Week 2.** In the 2nd week, you consume the same foods in the 20-hour period but you can start adding fat and protein in the 4-hour eating window period. Include nuts like almonds and macadamia nuts, chicken, salmon, tuna, tofu, mushrooms. You are aiming to improve your body's ability to utilize fat for energy.
- **Week 3.** In the 3rd week, the foods allowed during the 20-hour period remain the same but in the 4-hour eating window, you can have 1–2 higher-carb days and 1–2 lower-carb days over the course of a week. By doing this, you will help your body to utilize carbs to produce the energy you need.

Once the 3 phases are completed, they can be repeated, or you can stick with the 20:4 timing and focus on a higher protein, lower-carb pattern based on your personal needs.

I recommend this form of fasting for people who have tried other forms of IF already. Nutritionally speaking, it can be difficult to consume all the nutrients your body needs in this 20:4 version. And this will ultimately have an impact on energy levels and can lead to fatigue and high irritability. Other types of IF might be more beneficial to start with.

The Warrior Diet

Time Schedule	Monday	Tuesday	Wednesday	Thursday	Friday	Saturday	Sunday
Midnight 4 am 8 am 12 pm	Fast or Eat a small amount of fruits or vegetables	Fast or Eat a small amount of fruits or vegetable	Fast or Eat a small amount of fruits or vegetable	Fast or Eat a small amount of fruits or vegetable	Fast or Eat a small amount of fruits or vegetable	Fast or Eat a small amount of fruits or vegetable	Fast or Eat a small amount of fruits or vegetable
4pm – 8 pm	Large meal in 4 a hour eating window	Large meal in 4 a hour eating window	Large meal in 4a hour eating window	Large meal in 4 a hour eating window	Large meal in 4 a hour eating window	Large meal in 4 a hour eating window	Large meal in 4 a hour eating window
8 pm Midnight	Fast	Fast	Fast	Fast	Fast	Fast	Fast

Schedule is indicative and can be adjusted based on your daily routine

CHAPTER 6:

HOW TO START

So, if you are new to IF the question is how to get started. We described in a previous chapter the most popular IF methods, but really the most successful diet is the one you can stick to and the one that suits your lifestyle better. Keep reading for tips, advice, and how you can incorporate an IF schedule into your routine.

Create a Monthly Calendar

On a calendar, highlight the days on which you wish to fast, depending on the type of fast you have committed yourself to. Record a start and end time on your fasting days so you know in the days leading up to your fast day what time you plan to begin and finish.

Tick off your days; this will keep you motivated and on track!

Record Your Findings

Create a journal for your fasting journey. 1–2 days before the time you start the intermittent fasting, undertake to do your measurements. Weigh yourself first thing in the morning, after you have gone to the restroom, and before breakfast. Also, do not weigh yourself wearing heavy items as they may affect the outcome of the scale. Measure your height as this figure is related to your BMI (body mass index) result.

Record the measurements around your hips and stomach area, if you wish, you can also measure your upper thighs and arms.

Take a photo of yourself and place it into the journal too; this is not to discourage you but to keep you focused on why you began this journey. Jot down all of these findings and update them weekly in the journal.

A journal is also the perfect way to express how you are feeling and, of course, what you are most thankful for. A journal is an important way in which to track not just the physical aspects of the diet but also the mental aspects, too. Never doubt yourself; your journal should be a safe space for you to congratulate and to motivate yourself. Leave all the negative thoughts at the door!

Plan Your Meals

The easiest way to stick to any eating program is to plan your meals; 500 calorie meals tend to be simple and easy to create but there are also many other more complex recipes for those who wish to spice things up. Who knows, perhaps you stumble across a meal you wish to eat outside of your fasting days.

It is recommended that you cook your meals the day before your fast days; doing this helps you stay committed to the fast and limits food wastage.

Initially, and in the first few weeks, it is suggested that you keep your meal preparation and recipes simple, so as not to overcomplicate the whole process. This also allows you to get used to counting your calories and knowing which foods work to keep you fuller versus those that left you feeling hungrier earlier than later. Be sure to include your meal plan in your journal and on your calendar.

Reward Yourself

On the days where you return to normal eating, it is important to reward yourself. A slight prize goes a long way in reminding yourself and your brain that what you are doing has merit and that it should be noticed.

A reward should cater to one of our primal needs; these needs include:

- Self-actualization
- Safety needs
- Social needs
- Esteem needs

Have a block of chocolate or buy yourself a new item of clothing to do anything that makes your heart happy!

Curb Hunger Pains

Initially, you will feel more discomfort when hungry but these feelings will pass. If you do find yourself craving something, sip on black tea or coffee to help you through your day. Coffee is known to alleviate the feelings of being hungry; if you must add sweetener, do so at your discretion. Just remember that some sweeteners can cause the opposite effect and make you feel hungry.

Stay Busy

Keeping busy means that the mind does not have time to dwell on your current state of affairs, especially if you find yourself reaching for a snack bar or cookie.

It is also wise to be implementing some sort of physical activity, even on your fasting days. A 20-minute walk before ending your fasting period will do wonders to help you reach the final stages of the fasting period. It can also lift your mood once you are feeling upset or anxious.

Practice Mindful Eating

As mentioned, we are inclined to eat for all sorts of reasons; happy, sad, it does not matter. The problem is that these feelings related to food become habitual, so we aren't really hungry but because we feel good or even off, we seek to tuck into something delicious. The art of eating mindfully is to not allow these habits to master your life. The concept is simple: teach yourself to look at something, for instance, a piece of cake, and think, "Do I really need it or do I want it for other reasons?" You could decide to have 1–2 bites and leave the rest, but you may be less inclined to eat the whole slice (or whole cake) if you think mindfully about it. The art of mindful eating is to revel in the food placed before you. Pay attention to colors, textures, and tastes. Savor each bite, even when eating an apple. Your brain gradually begins to rewire itself when it comes to food and when it needs or wants something.

Practice mindful eating by:

- Pay consideration to where your food comes from.
- Listen to what your body is telling you; stop eating when you are full.
- Only eat when your body indicates you to do so; when your stomach growls or if you feel faint or if your energy levels are low.
- Pay attention to what is both healthy and unhealthy for you.
- Consider the environmental impact our food choices make.
- Every time you take a bite of your meal, set your cutlery down.

Practice Portion Control

Controlling portion sizes can be difficult for most; society has also regulated us to what we think is the size of an average portion should be and we have access to supersizing meals too, which does not help those struggling to maintain weight. In 1961, Americans consumed 2,880 calories per day; by 2017, they were consuming 3,600 calories, which is a 34% increase and an unhealthy one at that. To help you navigate how to better portion your food, consider trying the following: when dishing up your food, try the following trick. Half your plate should consist of healthy fruits and/or vegetables, one quarter should be made up of your starches such as potatoes, rice, or pasta, and the remaining quarter should be made up of lean meats or seafood.

Alternatively, try the following:

- Dish up onto a smaller plate or into a smaller bowl.
- Say no to upsizing a meal if offered.
- Buy the smaller version of the product if available or divide the servings equally into packets.
- Eat half a meal at the restaurant and take the remaining half to enjoy the following day instead.
- Go to bed early; it will stop any after-dinner eating.

INTERMITTENT FASTING FOR WOMEN OVER 50

Get Tech Savvy

Modern-day society has plenty to offer in terms of the apps we can use to help determine the steps we take, the calories we burn, the calories found in our foods, as well as research, information, and motivation for lifestyle changes, especially diets and exercise. The list is endless. There are numerous apps on the market at this time that can help you track your progress with regard to fasting.

The best IF apps currently (at the time of writing), and in no particular order are:

- Zero
- Fast Habit
- Body Fast
- Fasting
- Vora
- Ate Food Diary

Life Fasting Tracker

Make use of your mobile device to set reminders for yourself of when to eat, what to eat, and when your fast days are. It works especially well when using it to set reminders for when you should drink water, particularly for those who find it hard to keep their fluids up.

62 | P a g .

Making the Change

Understand that intermittent fasting is not a diet; it is a lifestyle, an eating plan that you are in control of, and one that is easy to perfect. Before you know it, fasting will become second nature.

When to Start?

Begin today, not tomorrow or after a particular event or gathering. Once you have picked the fast that best suits you, begin with it immediately. Never hold off until a specific day; once you begin, you will gain momentum and it will become something that is part of your day, like many other things that fill up your day. No sweat there!

Measure Your Eating

3 days before you fast, it would be wise to begin to lessen the amount of food you are eating or dishing up less. This helps your body begin to get used to the idea that it doesn't need a whole bowl of food to get what it needs nor to feel full.

Keep Up Your Exercise Plan

If you have a pre-existing exercise regime, do not alter it anyway. Simply carry on the way you were before fasting. If you are new to working out, start with short walks now and again, extending the time you walk. For example, take a 5-minute walk, and the next day, change the time to 10 minutes of walking.

Stop, Start, Stop

Fast for a period of hours, and then eat all your calories during a certain number of hours. Consider this as a training period.

Do Your Research

Read up as abundant as you can about IF. This way you will put to rest any uncertainties you might have and will get introduced to new ways of getting through a fasting day. Check out recipes that won't make you feel like a rabbit having to chomp on carrots all day if you are stuck with ideas of what to eat.

Have Fun

Have fun, and see what your body can do, even over 50. It is significant to distinguish that just because you are a certain age doesn't mean you are incapable of pursuing a new lifestyle change. Reward yourself when it is due, track your progress, adjust where there is a need, and get your beauty sleep. This is another secret to achieving overall wellness and happiness.

Know Your BMI

The body mass index (BMI) is a measure that helps you understand if your weight is healthy. Your BMI is based on the measurements of your weight and height; thus, you can easily control your body mass index, or BMI as it is more commonly known.

In total, there are 4 categories that an individual can fall into based on this figure. That is underweight, healthy, overweight, and obese. The concept is simple: our BMI gives us quantifiable amounts when comparing our height with our fat, muscles, bones, and organs.

How to Calculate Your BMI

To calculate your BMI divide your weight (pounds) by your height (inches) squared and multiply by 703.

Or you can use one of the many online calculators available on the internet.

As soon as you have calculated your BMI, you can compare it to the body mass index chart to determine which category you are classed into.

CLASS	YOUR BMI SCORE
Underweight	Less than 18.5 points
Normal weight	18.5–24.9 points
Overweight	25–29.9 points
Class 1—Obesity	30–34.9 points
Class 2—Obesity	35–39.9 points
Class 3—Extreme obesity	+40 points

CATHERINE LOGAN

CHAPTER 7:

DOS AND DON'TS ABOUT INTERMITTENT FASTING

S o, by now, you must be feeling ready to start your intermittent fasting journey. Keep reading for some dos and don'ts that will help you stay committed to your plan and make some healthy lifestyle changes.

The Dos

Regular contact with your doctor is an essential part of intermittent fasting. Try always to follow your doctor's suggestions and avoid using your own ideas, which can lead to harmful side effects. Ask your doctor to analyze your body weight and calorie intake so that you can adopt the right fasting plan.

Plan your fast schedule. Those who do not plan will fail. There are so many different IF methods available that those who are unaware of them might not be able to get the most out of fast. It is advisable that you have a plan before proceeding with fasting. Also, decide when you want to start fasting and how long you will be fasting for.

You don't want to become a cactus! Stay hydrated. Make sure you keep drinking water while limiting your calorie intake. Drinking water will cleanse your body and cleanse the blood vessels.

Fruits. If you cannot drink water in sufficient quantities, for some reason, try to eat fruits that have low sugar content such as cranberries and grapefruits, and remove unhealthy fat from your diet. They also contain a large amount of water. Apart from water, tea and black coffee are good add-ons to keep you hydrated.

Check your body's reactions closely. Try to track your body weight on a weekly basis as this will help you make a comparison and take decisions accordingly. Many people feel uncomfortable and tired when they first try IF.

Just make sure you don't lose weight by over-doing it. You might know someone who started to do IF and then became anorexic.

Fast to the degree that you could comfortably complete your daily work. Sometimes we tend to overdo fasting and this has a big effect on our daily activities.

Fasting can impact your intake of nutrients. Eat fruits that have great quantities of vitamins and minerals together with supplements. Vitamins will not break you fast but consider the time you take them. Some might irritate an empty stomach while others work best when consumed with food. Avoid products that are artificially sweetened.

Relax and enjoy the process. IF is not a dieting plan, it's an eating plan. There is no need to make the fasting days more demanding than the eating days. It's just a change in how much you're eating. Nothing more.

Start slow. To go from having 5–6 meals daily to eating only once a day can lead to very dire results. Apart from being harmful to your health, massive abrupt changes are hardly sustainable.

After confirming that IF is suitable for your health, the next thing to do is planning how to ease into the habit. In other words, before you fully implement any intermittent fasting regimen, it is a good practice to first test the waters, so to speak, with a less strict form of fasting. By doing this, it will help your body acclimate to the changes before going into the proper regimen.

Don't fuss over what you can eat. One common mistake people make when fasting is obsessing over the fasting hours and what to eat when they are finally allowed. You don't have to worry about what other people do. The important thing is what's comfortable for you. Of course, if your fasting window is too small, you are not likely to see any result. Also, don't get too tied up in every little detail of IF. For example, you don't have to become too worried because you missed a day.

Remember that intermittent fasting should be a lifestyle change if you want to continue to reap the benefits. And for a lifestyle change to be sustainable, you must be able to adapt and use it in a way that even if you face challenges, you will work your way around it somehow. Missing a day or cutting your fast short for reasons beyond your control shouldn't get you worked up and worrying about whether you can do the entire plan. Don't give up.

Again, some people focus too much on what they can eat or not eat. For example, "Can I add just a little butter or cream?" "Would it hurt to eat this type of food during the fasting window?" If your focus is on what you can have or eat while you are fasting, you are giving your attention to the wrong things and putting your mind in an unhelpful state. Give your mind the right focus by concentrating on doing a good, clean, fast, and try to consume only water, tea, or coffee during the window.

Give the calorie restriction a rest. Remember that IF is different from dieting. Your focus should be on eating healthily during your eating window or eating days instead of focusing on calorie restriction.

Even if you are fasting for weight loss, don't obsess over calories. Following a fasting regimen is enough to take care of the calories you consume. It is absolutely unnecessary to engage in a practice that can hurt your metabolism. Combining IF with eating too little food in your eating window because you are worried about your calorie intake can cause problems for your metabolism.

One of the major reasons that people push themselves into restricting calories while fasting is their concern for rapid weight loss. You need to be wary of any process that brings about drastic physical changes to your body in very short amounts of time. While it is okay to desire quick results, your health and safety are more important. When you obsess or worry that you are not losing weight as quickly as you want, you are not helping matters. Instead, you are increasing your stress level, and that is counterproductive. You are already taking practical steps toward losing weight by intermittent fasting. So why would you want to undo your hard work by unnecessary worrying? Simply focus on following a sustainable intermittent fasting regimen and let go of the need to restrict your calorie intake. Intermittent fasting will give your body the right number of calories it needs if you do it properly.

Watch electrolytes. Your body's electrolytes are compounds and elements that occur naturally in body fluids, blood, and urine. They can also be ingested through drinks, foods, and supplements. Some of them include magnesium, calcium, potassium, chloride, phosphate, and sodium. Their functions include fluid balance, regulation of the heart and neurological function, acid-base balance, oxygen delivery, and many other functions. It is important to keep these electrolytes balanced. But many people who practice fasting tend to neglect this and run into problems. Here is a common notion: "Don't let anything into your stomach until the end of your fast," even those just starting to fast know it doesn't work that way, and they tend to forget or fully stay away from liquids during their fasting window. When you lose too much water from your body through sweating, vomiting, and diarrhea, or you don't have enough water in your body because you don't drink enough liquids, you increase the risk of electrolyte disorders. It is not okay to drink tea or black coffee throughout the morning period of your fast window. You will wear down if you do not drink enough water. The longer you fast without water, the higher your chances of flushing out electrolytes and running into trouble. You can end up raising your blood pressure, develop muscle twitching and spasms, fatigue, fast heart rate or irregular heartbeat, and many other health problems. In contrast, drinking too much water can also tip the water-electrolyte balance. What you want to do is to drink adequate amounts of water and not excess water, whether you are fasting or not.

Break your fast gently. It is okay to feel very hungry after going for a long time without food, even if you were drinking water all through the fasting window. This is particularly true for people who are just starting with fasting. But don't let the intensity of your hunger push you to eat. You don't want to force food hurriedly into your stomach after going long without food, or you might hurt yourself and experience stomach distress. Take it slow when you break your fast. Eat light meals in small portions first when you break your fast. Wait for a couple of minutes for your stomach to get used to the presence of food again before continuing with a normal-sized meal. The waiting period will douse any hunger pangs and remove the urge to rush your meal. For example, break your fast with a small serving of salad and wait for about 15 minutes. Drink some water and then after about five more minutes, you can eat a normal-sized meal.

The first meal of the eating window is key. Breaking your fast is a crucial part of the process because if you don't get it right, it could quickly develop into unhealthy eating patterns. When you break your fast, it is important to have healthy foods around to prevent grabbing unhealthy feel-good snacks. Make sure what you are eating in your window is not a high-sugar or high-carb meal. I recommend that you consider breaking your fast with something that is highly nutrient-dense such as a green smoothie, protein shake, or a healthy salad. As much as possible, avoid breaking your fast with foods from a fast-food restaurant. Eating junk foods after your fast is a quick way to ruin all the hard work you've put in during your fasting window. If, for any reason, you can't prepare your meal, ensure that you order very specific foods that will complement your effort and not destroy what you've built. Although IF is not dieting and so, does not specify which foods to eat, limit, and completely avoid, it makes sense to eat healthily. This means focusing on eating a balanced diet, such as:

- o Whole grains.
- o Fruits and vegetables (canned in water, fresh, or frozen).
- o Lean sources of protein (lentils, beans, eggs, poultry, tofu, and so on).
- o Healthy fats (nuts, seeds, coconuts, avocados, olive oil, olive, and fatty fish).

Find a worthy goal. First things first; find a goal that is worth pursuing, or else you will drop the idea at the first sign of resistance. If you don't have a goal that represents a strong ideal, it won't be long before you start telling yourself, "I think I've passed the stage of such childishness." And yes, many women start a new lifestyle change for reasons that they can't keep up when things get tough. For example, the desire to look like models on TV, or social media makes losing weight feel socially acceptable and ok to keep up with trends that can be harmful. These reasons are not enough to keep anyone committed to a full lifestyle change and few wonder why so many people with goals are quick to jump from one lifestyle to another.

The Don'ts

To optimize the intermittent fasting effects, stay away from the things below.

Don't go into intermittent fasting because it is the thing to do at the moment. Instead, look for inspiring goals such as:

- o Staying fit, young, and healthy.
- o Improving your cognitive or brain functions.
- o Improving your overall vitality and increase energy levels.
- o Balancing hormones, especially during menopausal or post-menopausal stages of life.
- o Improving your overall health, thereby increasing longevity.

Does any of these sound good to you? Surely at this stage of your life, you are aware of the inherent risks of doing something merely because others are doing it too. That type of motivation will fail you.

Do not take too much before fasting. According to experts, heavy meals before fasting is strongly discouraged. It can harm your health, especially your stomach, due to the slow-burning nutrition in heavy or oily food.

Experts warn against fasting in conditions of health such as diabetes, cancer, and pregnancy. These conditions must be followed by precise steps. Consultation with a doctor is important for people with these health situations.

Do not be stressed out. Stress can increase your body's cholesterol level. Fasting will not work if excessive stress levels are induced in the body. Yoga and deep breathing are good practices for stress relief.

Don't do hard workouts. Yoga and jogging are always recommended to do during fasting. Remember that in the fasting state your energy level is lower. It goes without saying, therefore, that in this state you don't want to lift too much weight or run a marathon. Be comfortable with a lighter workout.

CHAPTER 8:

COMMON MISTAKES

Fasting is not generally seen as a diet but rather as a specific lifestyle and recommended eating schedule. This type of eating plan has gained enormous notoriety as of late, particularly for women over 50. As we have seen, you may fast for 16 hours and eat during an 8-hour window. This is the 16:8 plan and is commonly seen as the standard IF plan. A few people follow the alternate day plan, with low-calorie intake on one day and the usual amount the following. Whatever plan you choose to follow, when your goal is to get in shape, intermittent fasting is famous for one peculiar characteristic: it only works when done correctly.

There are a few potential health benefits when following intermittent fasting. Among them, it is the decreased danger of malignant growth, diabetes, and heart disease. Fasting can trigger autophagy, which is known to help with dementia. Regardless of whether you utilize one or another type of intermittent fasting, it is critical to avoid the traps that can undermine your endeavors. Below are a few intermittent fasting mistakes a lot of people make especially in the beginning:

Looking for Results Too Fast

You are preparing to begin something new, and you are eager to receive all the rewards as fast as could be. It is just normal that you are excited about this new lifestyle and you want to fully dive into it. Nevertheless, attempting to immediately get such a large number of improvements too early may disrupt your efforts.

The key is to begin gradually by including a couple of changes one after another. For instance, if you have chosen to do 2 500-calorie days every week while having a regular number of calories the other five; consider beginning with only 1 500-calorie day. After a couple of weeks, you can feel more confident including the 2nd day into your weekly schedule.

Slow and steady wins the race. This is an adage that we have all heard, but most of us do not believe it. We want fast results, and for this, we are ready to jump. However, this is not how the body works. Your body travels very slowly. You need time to adapt to any positive or negative change, and the same happens with intermittent fasting. If you want to succeed with this process, you must make sure you complete all the steps for a while. You have to allow your body some time to change and adapt. There are habits of decades that need to change, and sometimes it can be difficult for your body. If you want to adapt to change well, you shouldn't try to rush the process. Fasting in men and women is completely different. Men have a very resistant system and are not affected by a slightly extended rapid program. This is not the case for women. If you try to shake the system a little harder, this can negatively affect your health. Your hormonal system can change, and normalization can take a long time. A woman's body responds very differently to stress, and as a result, a woman needs to be vigilant and careful. Start with the simplest process and give your body time to adapt to small breaks. Once you are accustomed to a certain amount of break, try to stretch it a bit slowly. Always go step by step, and you will get to your goal easily and without unnecessary difficulties.

Confusing Thirst with Hunger

Not drinking enough water can make you hungry, and it is anything but difficult to sometimes confuse thirst with hunger.

People get a great deal of water from the foods they eat. Worldwide Food Information states that 20% of the water our bodies use originates from food. This implies that in case you are not eating for a few hours you will have to drink around 20% more water than usual to compensate for any shortfall.

We know that drinking water is fundamental for overall health, of course, yet it is even more significant when you are fasting. Why? Because most of the time we feel hungry we are actually dehydrated.

Can you imagine how your hunger might be influenced by lack of water when you are trying to go through the main part of the day without eating?

Fortunately, this is very simple to evade!

Sneaking extra water into your day is as simple as making a couple of basic changes.

Some people are truly bored with drinking plain water. Trust me, one thing that may be a great idea is to add a couple of Mio Drops (or other water enhancers) to water. It will have a tremendous effect!

In case you do not know them, Mio Drops are zero-calorie, zero-carb, and sugar-free water enhancers.

Eating Unhealthy Foods

Since IF is not generally a diet plan, there are not many foods that are "forbidden." This can lead numerous individuals to fall into the snare of a binge on junk food the moment their fast is up and the eating time opens. Try not to make a habit of unhealthy eating thinking that fasting will compensate for it.

Make a rundown of all the healthy foods you do appreciate. Do ordinary shopping for food and try to stick to your food decisions. While fulfilling your hunger with not exactly healthy snacks sometimes can be all right. But for ideal health and weight-loss achievement, it is important to eat as healthy as possible under the circumstances. Eating the right foods is vital to taking advantage of any weight loss plan. Foods rich in calcium, protein, and vitamin B-12 should be high on your grocery list, particularly for women over 50. This is because these nutrients help to keep the brain healthy while managing depression, balancing moods, and staving off cognitive decline.

The best way to overcome this trick is to have a very balanced meal. Your meals should be high in fat, moderate in protein, and low in carbohydrates. Before you begin to question the credibility of this suggestion, I would like to clarify some misconceptions: fat is not bad, but there is a popular misconception that eating fat is bad. Fat is the cornerstone of life. It plays an important role. Our bodies cannot function without fat.

Trans or low-quality fats that we get in processed foods are bad. Fat itself is a form of compact energy. Our body does not classify food as fat, protein, or cholesterol. Everything you eat is transformed and divided into calories. This means that fat would also be converted to glucose, and this would happen with carbohydrates. The advantage of eating fat is that you can eat more calories in a single meal than carbohydrates. Fat is very compact and has almost twice the calories per gram of carbohydrates. So, if you get 8 calories per gram of carbohydrates, you will get 16 fats. Protein is also heavier and has more calories than carbohydrates. This means that if you follow a diet high in fat and low in carbohydrates, you can get more calories. It also means that even if you eat fewer meals a day, you will not have a shortage of energy. It is very important to select high-quality fats. The same goes for proteins.

You can get protein from animals and cereals, and it would help you build muscle and stay fit. The biggest advantage of having a diet high in protein and low in carbohydrates is that it doesn't make you feel hungry very often. The fat and protein content in your meals would help you easily switch from one meal to another without addressing the need for snacks. Diets rich in fats and proteins also contain many minerals and vitamins. However, most minerals, vitamins, and fiber must be obtained from carbohydrates. You should consume many green leafy vegetables, salads, whole foods. The green leaves are bulky and do not weigh much. They don't add too many calories to your system, but they provide most of the vitamins, minerals, phytonutrients, antioxidants, and trace elements your body needs.

They are rich in fiber and, therefore, keep the digestive system healthy and also improve immunity. If you ignore your health, your weight will return faster than you can lose. People who lose weight drastically without a solid foundation can become sick and unhealthy. Always be mindful of the macronutrients that you consume and the calories that you take in. Do not consume anything within 30 minutes before going to sleep, as this will impede the natural process your body undergoes while asleep.

Keep your insulin levels low by not eating too many carbs or sugars and taking in protein before bed. Keep hydrated with a general gallon of water a day, and drink coffee early in the morning or late at night to keep alert during daylight hours.

Trying to Stick to the Wrong Plan

There are many different approaches to put IF into your daily schedule. For instance, if your fasting plan includes not eating from 8 p.m. until early afternoon every day and you have a challenging activity that begins right in the first part of the day, this is most likely not the correct plan for you.

What works for one person, may not necessarily fit in for another one. To get the most rewards of IF, you should take your time to thoroughly analyze different types of plans. It is all right if it takes a little longer to find out the plan that best works for you.

Working Out Too Much or Too Little

It is critical to remain as dynamic as possible, but you would prefer not to overdo it, especially during your fasting times. A few newbies may feel overwhelmed, beginning to follow a new eating schedule, and may overlook exercise altogether. Others might be so enthusiastic that they end up overdoing it.

It is a smart thought to pick a moderate exercise schedule, particularly when beginning. Strolling the pooch for twenty minutes or riding your bicycle to work are simple approaches to add moderate exercise to your customary calendar.

Misunderstanding Real Hunger Signs

Perhaps the best thing that I have learned from my IF test is that the body does not need any fuel to function. It can burn fat for a long time before it starts to break down muscle. This means that you can forgo breakfast and lunch for 16 hours, never feel hungry, and then eat dinner without overeating because your body's been burning fat all day (and evening, too!).

No doubt, your stomach may be growling, and you may desire something yummy.

Yet, you are not really hungry.

Also, it may be wonderful to binge with your family or friends and enjoy the social part of feasting.

Yet, again, you are not really hungry.

IF will teach you that if you stand by fasting long enough, more often than not, your "hunger" will blur generally in no more than five or ten minutes.

It most likely already happened without you noticing or giving it a particular thought.

How many times at work you were planning to go to eat, then some last-minute rush job showed up, and one hour or two passed by, while you overlooked your stomach's protest?

What before looked like the most urgent priority, eating, was overshadowed by something new that popped up. And you survived!

In any case, yielding and eating too early is one of the serious mix-ups with IF. Think that simply drinking some water and allowing ten minutes to pass by will usually calm down your appetite.

Try not to break your IF plan before you even begin.

Try not to easily give in to bogus hunger!

Using Intermittent Fasting as a Justification to Overeat

One of the most harmful IF mistakes is giving in to the temptation and say, "What the heck, I've starved myself throughout all the day, I deserve to reward myself for supper!"

and then diving into a crazy feast of junk food bombing yourself with unhealthy stuff.

Please don't be that woman.

You would feel hopeless, and most likely put on weight.

We don't want that.

In spite of the fact that, actually, IF is not a diet because it does not confine what you eat, it is yet critical to settle on healthier food decisions. You want, most of all, to have a healthy relationship with your food and your body.

You can absolutely overeat and put on weight even by eating just once per day, in the event you are eating a bigger number of calories than your body consumes.

While you do not need to be an absolute stickler and there is space for adaptability, still, be shrewd.

Help yourself out and do not go crazy during your eating window.

Not Eating Enough

If you have yet to attempt IF, the risk of not eating enough during eating times may appear to be illogical.

Actually, for some people, not eating for a particularly long period of time, it's not unusual to become less hungry.

In some cases, fasting can thoroughly kill your appetite.

Unless you are deliberately doing a total fast (not suggested if not under medical control), however, it is anything but a good idea to decide not to eat enough.

If you do not eat sufficiently for too long, you can easily wreck your digestion and unbalance your hormones.

Moreover, you will deny your body fundamental nutrients, which can help to avoid health issues that are far more important than the loss of a couple of additional pounds.

Failing to Plan Your Meals in Advance

While calorie tallying is not important (however, truly, you will show more signs of improvement results if you do it), carefully planning and thinking about what you will eat when your eating period arrives is a great IF hack.

This will allow you not to have to improvise when you are finally going to sit down at the table.

Perseverance Is the Key

Impatience is a big problem in people struggling with weight. Most people trying to lose weight have already faced disappointments with other weight-loss tactics and therefore want to see the results quickly. They are not ready to wait long for the results. This is a point where problems can occur. IF is a wonderful process, but it does not work by magic. The results might take time to arrive. You will have to work with patience and not lose hope when results are slow. It is not a process that works overnight. A leap of faith will be required, and you will need to devote your time and energy.

Don't Frame Unrealistic Expectations

We all like to dream big, and that is a good thing. However, we must also remain based on reality. This will help to accept the facts and save many disappointments. Many times, we are so caught up in unreal expectations that we don't recognize the gifts we receive. If your goal is weight loss, think about the amount of time you are ready to devote, the distances you can travel, and the medical conditions you face. Without considering all these facts, expecting a complete makeover would be absurd and your expectations would overshadow the results. It is important to stay realistic.

CHAPTER 9:

WHAT TO EAT AND WHAT TO AVOID

What to Eat

Berries

Berries are very healthy, incredibly flavorful, and much lower in calories and sugar than you might think! Their tart sweetness can bring a smoothie to life, and they make a delicious snack on their own without any help from things like cream or sugar.

Cruciferous Vegetables

These are vegetables like cabbage, Brussels sprouts, broccoli, and cauliflower. These are beautiful additions to your diet because they're packed with vital nutrients and with fiber that your body will love and use quickly!

Eggs

Eggs are such a great addition to your diet because they're packed to the gills with protein, you can do just about anything with them, they're easy to prepare and they can pair with just about anything. They're an excellent protein source for salads, and they're right on their own as well.

Fish

In particular, whitefish is typically very lean, but fish like salmon that have a little bit of color in them are packed with protein, fats, and oils that are great for you. They're good for your brain and heart health, and there's a massive array of delicious things you can do with them.

Healthy Starches Like Individual Potatoes (With Skins!)

In particular, red potatoes are excellent to eat, even if you're trying to lose weight because your body can use those carbs for fuel, and the skins are packed with minerals that your body will enjoy. A little bit of potato here and there can do good things for your nutrition, but they are also a great way to make you feel like you're getting a little more of those fun foods that you should cut back on.

Legumes

Beans, beans, the magical fruit. They're packed with protein, and the starch in them makes them stick to your ribs without making you pay for it later. They're lovely in soups, salads, and just about any other meal of the day that you're looking to fill out. By adding beans to your regimen, you might find that your meals stick with you a little bit longer and leave you feeling more satisfied than you thought possible.

Nuts

I know you've heard people talking about how a handful of almonds makes a great snack, and if you're anything like me, you've always had kind of a hard time believing it. Nuts, as it turns out, have a good deal of their healthy fats in them that your body can use to get through those rough patches and, while they are not the most satisfying snack on their own, you might consider topping your salad with them for a little bit of crunch, or pairing them with some berries to make them a little more satisfying.

Probiotics Help Boost Your Gut Health

Having a happy gut often means that your dietary success and overall health will improve!

Vegetables That Are Rich in Healthy Fats

Not to sound topical or trendy, but avocados are a great example of a vegetable packed with healthy fats. Look for vegetables with fatty acids and a higher fat content, and you will find that if you add more of those into your regimen, you will get hungry less often.

Water, Water, Water, and More Water

No matter what you decide to add to or subtract from your regimen, stay hydrated. It will help digestive health and it will keep you from feeling slump or tired, and keep you also from getting too hungry. Add electrolytes where you need to, and don't be shy about bringing a bottle with you when you go from place to place. Stay hydrated!

What to Avoid

Grains

Whole grains may have their health benefits and be full of fiber but you can also get these nutrients elsewhere. The human diet does not require grain consumption. The truth is while grains may have some benefits, they are ridiculously high in both total and net carbohydrates, making them incompatible with the ketogenic diet.

Some people do try what is known as the targeted ketogenic diet, which is a version of the diet specifically designed for those who complete extended and strenuous workouts. With the targeted ketogenic diet, a person will consume a small serving of carb-heavy food, such as grains, for thirty to forty minutes before working out.

Sugary Fruits

Most fruits contain a high sugar content, meaning that they are also high in carbohydrates. The exception is that you can enjoy berries, lemons, and limes in moderation. Some people will also enjoy a small serving of melon as a treat from time to time, but watch your portion size as it can add up quickly!

Milk and Low-Fat Dairy Products

Sadly, milk is much higher in carbohydrates than cheese, with 1 glass of 2% milk containing twelve carbs, half of your daily total. Instead, choose low-carb and dairy-free milk alternatives such as almond, coconut, and soy milk. Also, you may consider using low-fat cheeses instead of full fat to reduce the saturated fats you are consuming.

Cashews, Pistachios, and Chestnuts

While you can enjoy nuts and seeds in moderation, keep in mind that nuts contain a moderate carbohydrate level and therefore should be eaten in moderation. However, some nuts including cashews, pistachios, and chestnuts are high in carbs and thus are better to be avoided.

If you want to enjoy nuts, you can fully enjoy almonds, pecans, walnuts, macadamia nuts instead.

Most Natural Sweeteners

While you can undoubtedly enjoy sugar-free natural sweeteners such as stevia, monk fruit, and sugar alcohols, you should avoid natural sweeteners that contain sugar. Suffice to say, and the sugar content makes these sweeteners naturally high in carbs. But not only that, but they will also spike your blood sugar and insulin.

Alcohol

Drinking alcohol during your fasting period will break your fast as it contains calories. However, you are allowed to drink alcohol in moderation during your eating window. Keep in mind though that alcohol contains calories and its consumption has been shown to block fat breakdown while also it might stimulate overeating which can lead to weight gain over time. So, please remember, if you do drink, stick to lower-alcohol wine and hard spirits and add some water to limit the intake of extra calories. Avoid sugary cocktails and instead drink dry wine, vodka, gin, or tequila.

Intermittent Fasting and the Keto Diet

What are the 2 hottest trends right now? IF and the keto diet. So, the question is, can you combine them?

With the ketogenic diet the majority of the calories you eat come from fat, while the rest come from a moderate amount of protein and a small number of carbs which essentially means saying hello to meat and eggs and bye-bye to fruits and pasta.

The idea with this high-fat, low-carb diet is to transition your body from burning glucose (or carbs) for fuel to burning fat for energy. This state as we mentioned earlier is called ketosis.

If you are on a keto diet and struggle to reach ketosis you might want to consider adding IF which may effectively jumpstart your process. How does it work? The keto diet increases levels of ketones in the body. During fasting ketones also increase. Combining them might allow your body to reach the ketosis stage faster than the keto diet alone.

Switching from glucose to fat as fuel is a big change. For this reason, if you consider combining both IF and keto diet you should always start with the keto diet to allow your body to adjust and then after a couple of months, you can consider layering with IF. Again, as mentioned many times in this book, before making any nutritional change, always consult with your doctor.

CHAPTER 10:

MAINTAINING WEIGHT

As soon as you have grasped your goal weight, you will want to keep a maintenance diet plan and keep your calories under control; at first, it may seem like hard work, but it eventually becomes second nature. Fasting should be on your list of things to do every now and then, or at least once a month.

If you keep fasting you will be able to navigate fasting times without too much hunger. If you keep eating food that keeps you fuller for longer and keeps you well hydrated, you will start to have more energy and feel healthier.

The problem of weight relapse is even more difficult than the initial weight loss. To be able to understand this topic we will also have to understand the issue of losing water weight.

What Is Water Weight?

We all are made up of water. A major portion of our weight comes from water. It runs in our veins in the form of blood. There is a lot of moisture in our tissues. Water is in our body in various forms.

However, our body also retains water in its actual form for various purposes. One of the most important functions is to regulate body temperature. You might have observed that people in good health feel less hot or cold as compared to other people who aren't in such good health. It happens because all healthy people have a lot of water in their bodies, regulating the temperature.

A part of the energy that we get through food is used for this purpose. The more well-fed or well-nourished and healthy we are, the more comfortable we are likely to feel. The reason is simple; your body will have ample energy to spare to make you feel comfortable.

The water that is used for this temperature regulation has its weight. That weight is called water weight.

What Leads to the Loss of Water Weight?

When you begin the process of losing weight, the first thing that you target is calorie intake. We are repeatedly told that if we eat more calories, we will get fat. Therefore, as per conventional wisdom, we begin by lowering our calorie intake.

The first impact of lower calorie intake is that it creates an energy deficit.

Before we move any further, you must understand the concept of basal metabolic rate or BMR. Our body has 2 kinds of energy needs:

- The constant energy need
- The variable energy need

The constant energy need is the fixed energy requirement of your body to run the crucial functions like blood circulation, the pumping of the heart, the functioning of the kidneys, the liver function, etc.

The body needs to run these processes all the time, even when the person is sleeping or in a medical coma. The energy demand created by such processes is called the BMR. It can be calculated by a specific mathematical formula that keeps into account your weight, height, gender, and other such things.

This is the minimum energy required by the body to survive even if you are not doing any physical activity. Even if you don't move a muscle, your body would need these many calories.

The variable energy need can vary depending upon the kind of physical activity undertaken by you. Energy needs to maintain an active lifestyle would be higher. The same would be lower for a person leading a sedentary lifestyle. In the same way, there are several processes that the body runs when it is in an energy surplus. Those processes have the end goal of providing you comfort. Regulating the body heat against outside temperature is one such comfortable energy expenditure.

Whenever you go on a calorie-restrictive diet, your body would need to cut energy. You can rely on the prudence of the body; it will always try to bring down the variable energy needs first.

When you lower your calorie intake, the body starts looking for areas to cut energy. The first thing to go is temperature regulation. As a result, your body starts dumping excess water rapidly.

If you have ever been on a calorie-restrictive diet, you would appreciate the fact that the weight loss in the initial period is rapid, and it starts plateauing after a few weeks. The reason is simple. Initially, your body is hoarding a lot of water and it starts dumping it rapidly and that's why you see a rapid weight loss. But once you have lost your water weight, the calorie restriction cannot help you with weight loss.

Why Calorie Restriction Is Ineffective in Actual Weight Loss

Most people believe that if they lower the calorie intake below a certain level, the body would start targeting its fat stores for energy. However, even you wouldn't do that in normal circumstances, if you know that there is going to be a shortage of something. Rationing is in our very nature.

When you lower your calorie intake, the body first tries to lower its variable energy needs. However, there is a limit to that. If you have an active lifestyle, even when your calorie intake is low, your variable energy needs would remain high. You may feel tired more often but you will still keep getting the required energy.

In such a case, the body would start to look for areas to lower its constant energy needs. When many animals go into hibernation, their heartbeats become slow. Their whole metabolic process slows down so that they can survive on the same amount of energy for much longer. The body starts doing the same with the BMR.

In the case of a strict calorie-deficient diet, you may feel tired more often. There can be a feeling of lethargy and unwillingness to do anything. All these are subtle hints being dropped by the body to lower the energy expenditure.

If you observe, until now there is no mention of the body making any effort to use the energy stored in the form of fat.

You must remember that the body would only come for stored energy only when the outside energy supply comes to a halt and not when it becomes low or slow.

This is the biggest reason people don't experience fat-burning by simply following a calorie-restrictive diet.

The diets can only be for a specific period. Once you get off a diet, you would have very strong food temptations. This leads to binge eating, and the weight comes back even faster than you had lost it.

The Reason for Weight Relapse

Most women think that if they don't eat too much, they won't face weight relapse. However, they get disappointed, and even with a very restricted calorie intake, they start experiencing weight gain. It is incorrect to think that you will only lose weight when you eat a lot. It is not the food but the amount of energy going inside you that will lead to weight gain. As soon as you resume eating the required number of calories, there is no need for the body to not begin the process of heat regulation. It begins retaining the water once again, and hence you see a rapid rise in your weight.

You must understand that weight lost or gained in a short period is water weight. It is not the weight lost by the body due to the burning of actual body fat.

Clean Food for a Clean Mindset

Clean eating is a concept whereby a person makes themselves aware of where the food came from and how it got to their plate. In other words, eating foods that are not processed, and contain no GMOs or pesticides. Food not only has to be cooked in cleaner, more natural ways, but it has to have been handled that way before it was bought, too.

Making the more natural and healthy choice when choosing your foods means cutting outboxed, packaged, processed, bagged, or artificially colored and flavored foods. Instead of going for the can of fruit choose the organic fresh fruit.

These foods are called whole foods and include fresh foods, whole grains, unrefined sugars, less dairy, and lower salt. All of which is a lot healthier reduces the risk of disease and improves a person's overall health. After a person becomes familiar with and used to fasting, they will want to make healthier choices as they start to feel cleaner on the inside.

At first, you may think it is quite the mission to make these choices but if you persevere and take the extra minute to read the back of a can or package you will notice all the added ingredients. Most of which you probably cannot even pronounce. You are making the effort to become healthier, lose weight, and feel better so go the extra mile and make those better food choices.

Once you have tasted the difference in whole foods over-processed, refined, and artificially grown, flavored, or colored you will naturally avoid them. Eating clean reprograms both your mind and body to want cleaner foods.

CHAPTER 11:

MYTHS ABOUT INTERMITTENT FASTING

Your Body Will Go Into Starvation Mode and Metabolism Will Slow Down

Truth: Your body won't enter starvation mode through IF. Skipping meals or acclimating to longer periods between meals where you don't eat won't make you starve. Your metabolism will not slow down and stop burning fat. Again, IF isn't about restricting calories but restricting the time in which calories are consumed. In fact, studies have shown that short-term fasts up to 48 hours increase your metabolic rate through the increase of norepinephrine in blood. Norepinephrine's role is to regulate metabolism and blood pressure.

You'll Lose Muscle

Truth: This is another misconception. Your body won't lose muscle through IF. When you fast, you turn to body fat and not muscle for energy needs. Doing a little exercise or workout will help you maintain your muscles and stay fit.

You'll Certainly Indulge During Eating Windows

Truth: While a few people will feel the need to indulge during eating windows, not every person will gorge

Your body will ask you to indulge because, in the beginning, it won't understand what is happening, however, after a short period of time it will adjust and so will your hunger.

There's Just a Single Method to Do IF

Truth: There is no right approach to practice IF, and part of the excellence of IF is that there are various techniques. There's no right technique for everybody, and there's no "best" strategy to make progress toward. Try whatever technique feels right and suits your lifestyle, and practice it for as long as you can! That is undeniably the best approach.

You'll Become Extremely Healthy and Fit by Fasting

Truth: IF is a change in your lifestyle. It does not work overnight and you will get the best results if you combine it with regular exercise and a healthy nutritious diet. Even though many studies have shown its benefits on health, it is certainly not a cure for all diseases.

It's For Everyone

Truth: IF became very popular in the past few years and is promoted as beneficial for all people. This is true in most cases and if you don't overdo it. However, there are certain groups of people that should steer clear. Children, pregnant women, and underweight people. These groups need to eat more and not restrict their calories. Also, people with high blood sugar should proceed with caution and medical supervision is essential.

CHAPTER 12:

HOW TO STAY MOTIVATED

D o you know what a fasting regime and New Year resolutions have in common? They start out great for a couple of months. The third month; some hitches here and there. By the 6–7th month, some people have issues remembering what their resolutions were in the first place.

If you have fallen by the wayside, you'll be relieved to know you're not alone. Even the most enthusiastic fitness gurus struggle sometimes to stay on course. If you have already missed a few steps, you can start all over again and get it right this time. Here are some tips which will help you stay motivated:

Get an Accountability Partner

Having someone alongside you with similar goals can keep you on course especially when you struggle to stay on track with exercise and healthy eating. With the internet, your accountability partner can even be in another continent. Having someone to hold your hand when you need it, to discuss challenges and frustrations, can really help you to succeed in achieving your goals. Motivation increases when knowing that someone will check on your progress. You can share tips, recipes, struggles but what is more interesting is that you might even develop a new friendship.

Keep Informed

How much do you know about IF? The more you know, the easier it will be for you to go through the process. Read blogs and watch videos to understand what other women, and indeed men have to say about fasting. This will also help you keep your expectations realistic. When it comes to weight loss, women can be impatient. A few days on a diet and you're already in front of the mirror looking for changes. Don't worry; we've all been there!

You know by now that IF is a way to lose weight fast; but how fast is fast? Getting the right information, especially from those who have gone through the same process already, will let you know what to expect, and you'll be better prepared to deal with any issues that may arise.

Set Goals with Rewards

Setting milestones with some goodies attached to them will keep you going even when your body and mind tell you otherwise. Keep in mind though that the reward, in this case, is not food-related.

Why can't you treat your sweet tooth as a reward? Well, to begin with, what you'd be saying to your mind is that the healthy foods you're eating are a punishment of sort, and only after eating them will you get some "good" food. Secondly, if you indulge in sugary and fatty treats, you'll only roll back on the gains already made. We don't want any of that, do we?

Your goal here is mainly weight loss, among other health gains. Once you've reached a goal of losing a certain number of pounds in a set time, you can treat yourself to a shopping trip for new clothes. Enjoy fitting in clothes that you would not have worn before. As you stare at yourself in the mirror and admire the new you, you'll be even more motivated to work towards your next goal.

Concentrate on Positive Feelings

How do you feel after shedding some pounds? I'm sure you're enjoying fitting into a smaller-size outfit, looking more presentable, feeling confident, being physically active without straining, and so on.

Let these feelings color your day. Every time a thought crops upon how hungry you are or how many foods you can no longer eat, remind yourself how dashing you look in that new dress.

Every time a negative feeling lingers, counter it with a positive thought and watch your energy revive.

Healthy-Eating Mind

Living healthy is choosing to be kind to your body, and knowing that it will remit the kindness right back. Think of your body for a moment as a separate entity from yourself. How would it feel when constantly being fed the wrong foods that bring you terrible effects? How would it feel to constantly be fed on too much food and you have to strain to digest? If your body could speak, it could possibly ask these questions.

Feed it the right foods, because it is the right thing to do. Give it just the right amount, without overloading it with unnecessary carbs, sugar, and fats. And give it a break from all the digesting work occasionally, who does not like a good rest?

Visualize the Future

Just picture how your future will turn out if you keep living this healthy lifestyle. You'll be disease-free, active, radiant, and energetic. You'll improve your longevity, enjoying a longer, fuller life.

What's the other side of the coin? A life with many health issues. I'm sure you know such people. They're no longer able to do the things they enjoy. Their activity level is largely reduced if not cut off altogether. They carry medicine wherever they go. Isn't the idea of such a life horrifying, especially in a case where different choices were all that was needed for a different turnout?

Choosing health is choosing life. If you still have the chance, this is an opportunity that you have to embrace. You work so hard to make sure your final days watch you age gracefully, don't let an unhealthy life take this dream away from you.

Join a Community of Like Minds

Thank God for the Internet; we can now form groups with people of similar interests even from different continents. Search the internet for women in intermittent fasting, and you should be able to find such groups. You can then exchange messages, photos, and videos of your progress. That only helps you stay consistent. Share experiences, tips, goals, recipes, survival tactics, and so on. Alone you can get discouraged and quit, but such a "healthy living family" will not let you fall by the wayside.

CONCLUSION

W ith intermittent fasting, changes occur in the body by promoting increased longevity, cellular repair, decreased inflammation, and changes in the hormonal control of body weight.

Only a single bout of fasting may have beneficial effects, but it is important to focus on finding a fasting method that you can sustain over the long run.

It could be easier for some people to follow an IF plan than a conventional "don't eat this or that" diet because it does not restrict the amount of food eaten. Based on each individual's needs, some may choose to layer their fasting technique with a food-specific diet. However, it is always best to consult with your doctor or a qualified healthcare professional before making dietary changes.

As we end this book please remember:

- Along with eating healthy, regular exercise is a must.
- Intermittent fasting could help you lose weight, but don't expect fat to magically melt off your body.
- Your intermittent fasting plan should be enjoyable because if you don't enjoy doing it then chances are you

will not stick to it and then you won't get the results that you want.

- Some people find that intermittent fasting helps them to maintain a healthy weight.

- Intermittent fasting should not be practiced by pregnant women or people who are seriously ill or suffering from a chronic illness like diabetes.

- Don't forget to drink lots of water every day when practicing intermittent fasting.

- Intermittent fasting can have health benefits, but it is important to remember that fasting is not a magic bullet that will cure any disease.

Now you understand what intermittent fasting is and how it can help you lose weight efficiently, safely, and comfortably. Intermittent fasting is so powerful because you can use it to restrict calories, induce ketosis, and activate the processes of autophagy

Thank you for making it through to the end of *Intermittent Fasting for Women Over 50*, let's hope it was enlightening and able to offer you all of the gears you need to attain your goals whatever they may be.

117 | P a g .

Printed in Great Britain
by Amazon